Fit Happens with Know Exercise!

28 Days of Success for Every Body

Stephanie Hilton Sewell

iUniverse, Inc.
New York   Bloomington

Fit Happens with Know Exercise!
28 Days of Success for Every Body

iUniverse books may be ordered through booksellers or by contacting:

iUniverse
1663 Liberty Drive
Bloomington, IN 47403
www.iuniverse.com
1-800-Authors (1-800-288-4677)

ISBN: 978-1-4502-1491-9 (sc)
ISBN: 978-1-4502-1493-3 (dj)
ISBN: 978-1-4502-1492-6 (ebk)

Library of Congress Control Number: 2010923262

Printed in the United States of America

iUniverse rev. date: 4/2/2010

Other products available from Stephanie Sewell at
www.StephanieSewell.com

5 STEPS to a Healthier You Exercise DVD
5 STEPS to a Healthier You - Kids Boot Camp Edition Exercise DVD
Cardio in 5—A four-disc Audio Cardiovascular Workout Program

This book is dedicated to my family, clients, and friends who have allowed me to inspire and motivate them to a healthier lifestyle. I would like to give special thanks to Mercedes Miller, Kondria Woods and Tina Parker for their guidance and direction during this journey.

Today is a New Day!
I will choose Success over Failure
Strength over Weakness!
I will Love my Body Nutritionally
Not Harm it Carelessly
Because Today is a New Day!

Stephanie Sewell

Contents

Introduction

Congratulations on taking the first step to a healthier you! I am Stephanie Sewell, speaker, teacher, empowerment coach, and personal trainer. I will share my workout and healthy eating secrets with you to help you make "fit happen with know exercise." What you hold in your hands is the ultimate daily fitness journal! All you need is a positive attitude and *Fit Happens with Know Exercise! 28 Days of Success for Every Body* (I will refer to this book as the *Fit Happens Journal* from this point), and you are ready to Get up ... Get Moving ... *and* Get Fit! My *Cardio in 5* Program and my *5 STEPS to a Healthier You* exercise DVD series are additional items available to help you reach a healthier you.

But first, here are the disclaimers. Be sure to consult your doctor prior to starting, changing, or altering your exercise and eating program. The information provided in this *Fit Happens Journal,* as well as in the *Cardio in 5,* and *5 STEPS to a Healthier You* DVD, is for general knowledge and should not to be used as a substitute for medical advice. Stephanie Sewell and StephanieSewell.com have documented the steps taken to get fit. This is Stephanie Sewell's personal exercise regimen and she has used the nutritional guidelines contained within to reduce overall body weight in preparation for fitness and pageant competitions. Stephanie Sewell, StephanieSewell.com, or other producers, personal trainers, and associates cannot be held liable for injury. Weight loss results are not typical, and there are no guarantees for body weight reduction.

Prior to beginning the workout recommendations of this *Fit Happens Journal,* check all equipment for defects before initiating each exercise session. Be sure to warm up and cool down at the beginning and end of every exercise session. Ensure complete recovery and sufficient rest between levels of intensity. Stop exercising immediately if you feel pain or discomfort from the movement. Also, stop exercising immediately if you cannot talk or if you feel dizzy. Discontinue the exercise when proper form cannot be maintained.

The foods listed are not federally endorsed and have not been tested for diagnosis, treatment, or prevention of any diseases.

My Reality Check

I had to drag myself out of bed. It was time to gain control over my life and my body. I had to unearth the old dreadful scale from the far corner of my closet so I could weigh myself. Before that could happen, I knew I had to empty my bladder and whatever else needed to be emptied before stepping on that scale. You've heard the old saying: weigh yourself on an empty stomach and with an empty bladder to see your true weight.

Since the beginning of our marriage, my husband and I had an agreement that we would let each other know when we noticed the other was moving in an unhealthy direction. He can tell when he sees the dimples in my butt! I can tell when I can no longer see his belt buckle. Imagine my surprise when my husband told me the previous night, just as we were turning in for the night, that I had a pumpkin butt… and it was *not* Halloween. I had to sleep with that knowledge. At first light of the next day, I knew it was time to get back to working out. Oh, I knew the time was coming, as I'd noticed that I gained every pound of my personal maximum weight. Every week, I would try on my clothes to see what would fit. I tried to blame the dry cleaners and the seamstress, claiming they were shrinking my clothes or not fitting them properly to my measurements. Ultimately, I had to agree with my husband once I saw the dimples for myself. And the scale read… "Unfit for you." I couldn't blame anyone except myself. Fortunately, there is no time to play the "blame game"… only time to work on a sound game plan.

I am a former Swimsuit Winner, State Pageant Competitor, National Fitness Competitor, and former NFL Cheerleader. I am a petite, thirty-something wife, mother, and entrepreneur. The reality check was found in my dimpled, pumpkin-shaped butt. That was my wake-up call. Thanks to the program I followed in my *Fit Happens Journal*, I am ready and able to share my success with others. I can honestly say that I practice what I preach!

In my preparation for a pageant, fitness competition, or a cheerleading event, I always made sure to research the event I was preparing for, execute with precision, and deliver a knock-out performance. Lately, I have allowed "LIFE" to get in the way. That's when:

> Little,
> Insignificant
> Factors
> Enter my world!

When that happens, I notice a change in my personal ABCs: my Attitude, Body Image, and the Calories I bring into my "LIFE."

The *Fit Happens Journal* had worked for me in the past, and I proudly put it to the test once again. This time, I am adding a twist! This program is a documentation of my personal experience—every step of the way—and is designed to be an interactive journal. Please start your day with this resource and design a program that will work for you! Albert Einstein once said, "The definition of insanity is doing the same thing over and over again and expecting different results." I am a firm believer that, once you decide you are sick and tired of being sick and tired, you will find strength within yourself to make a change. Now, get your pen or pencil out and keep reading! It is time for you to get with the *Fit Happens Journal!*

My Reality Check

Date: September 2008
Weight: Too Heavy for Me
Height: Petite

Measurements
Neck: Plump
Chest: Too Much Bounce
Waist (Circumference of Natural Curve): Love Handles on the Left and Right
Waist (Circumference from Belly Button): Muffin Top
Hips: Juicy
Upper Thigh (Widest Part): Loosey-Goosey
Arm (Circumference of Bicep): Jiggly-Wiggly

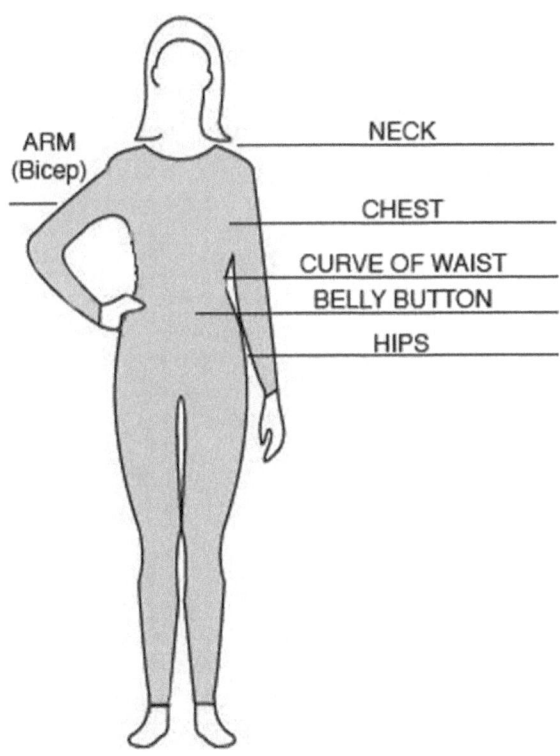

Week One

Why

Day #1

Your Reality Check

I'm so glad you are moving forward with the *Fit Happens Journal*. I hope my experience has given you the courage to complete Your Reality Check. In order to know where you are going, you have to know your personal starting point. Day #1 is all about you. This is *your* reality check.

Have you seen a picture that someone has taken of you and you didn't recognize yourself? I know I have. After seeing a recent picture from our vacation, I was upset with the person who took the picture for not telling me that I looked like that!

For Day #1, select someone to take your picture and your measurements. I would recommend you wear something fitted that you are comfortable wearing for this brief photo session. Also, I suggest the more skin you have showing, the better, so you can see your true starting point.

When having your picture and measurements taken, resist the temptation to hold in your stomach! Do not hold your breath! Do not wear baggy clothes! And, whatever you do, *do not skip* Day #1. This is the most important day!

It is time for you to see the *real you*! Trust me. My clients who opted to skip this initial step in their Fit Happens journey were later unhappy about not documenting their starting point. I would not want you to miss out on the joy this day will bring you when you reach your goal—especially when you are fit and trim and ready for your affair!

Items Needed

Pen/Pencil
Camera
Someone to Take Your Picture
Fitted Outfit
Measuring Tape
Scale
Date:
Weight:
Height:

Measurements (inches)

Neck:
Chest:
Waist (Circumference of Natural Curve):
Waist (Circumference from Belly Button):
Hips:
Upper Thigh (Widest Part):
Arm (Circumference of Bicep):

Stephanie Hilton Sewell

[Insert Photo Here]

Day #2

Plan to Have an Affair

I know ... you are wondering why this self-help exercise guide is talking about having an affair. At this point, you probably thought I would have jumped into telling you to run three miles and eat a selection of low-fat, low-calorie, no-taste foods for Day #2, right? Wrong! I'm a real person and I'm going to share things I have done to get my mind and body in sync to get fit.

Now, let's get back to your future affair! It all depends on you. I'm talking about setting goals and finding out what you must do to reach your goals. By having an affair, you are identifying some type of event that is important to you. The *Fit Happens Journal* will help you reach your goals, but you have to crystallize your goal and write it down in order to achieve it.

First, let's define an "affair." One dictionary meaning of an affair is "an event or occurrence that has been referred to or is known about." My definition of an affair is "something *big*!" It could be a wedding, a pageant, a high school class or family reunion, a trip, or a competition. It has to be a tremendous event where *you* stand in the spotlight! You're probably asking what I mean by that statement. If you are attending an event as a guest or the event is for someone else, it doesn't count. If the people in attendance really don't know you, or you are attending it with a friend, co-worker, or significant other, that doesn't count either.

If your ex or your companion's ex will be in attendance, then that would count as an affair! In all sincerity, I would like for your occasion to be something where you will be the center of attention. When all eyes are on you, you will be more focused on making sure you are prepared and ready for that attention.

Let me share an example of my affair with you. I am a former Carolina Panthers cheerleader, pageant winner, and fitness competitor. After getting married, I settled down on our cushy sofa and dug into generous helpings of chips and ice cream. One day, I realized I wanted to compete again, so I had an affair to prepare for. I set my sights on the Miss Fitness Universe Pageant. It was an event that I had some prior knowledge of, and I wanted to see if I had what it would take to make a comeback. Based on my background, experience, and work ethic, I believed I was ready to set the wheels in motion to move forward with my affair.

My question to you is this: are you choosing an affair that is good for you or good for someone else? I'm asking you that question because you will work harder for your own affair than for an affair that someone else wants you to have. When you are convinced by someone else to have an affair, you compromise your goals and values to satisfy someone else's desire. Not only are you pleasing someone else, you run the chance of losing yourself and losing your grip on your personal goals in the journey. So please ... *please* ... choose an affair wisely. Make sure that you are committed to *your* affair. You have to be willing to go the extra mile because, remember, it is *your* time to shine.

Items Needed

Pen/Pencil
Calendar

If you have decided to have an affair, and you are ready to prepare for the affair, then you should be willing to go the extra mile. Let's get started by writing some juicy details about the affair to make sure you will be prepared!

I, _____ will follow the program in the *Fit Happens with Know Exercise: 28 Days of Success for Every Body Journal (Fit Happens Journal)* to assist me in preparing for

_____

Please write some information about your affair here:

_____

(Your goal and/or your event and its date—for example, Family Reunion, Date)

    Did you choose a special occasion, vacation, reunion, or overall health? The choice is yours. And remember, it is something *big*! It could be a wedding, a pageant, a special trip, or a competition. It has to be a tremendous event where *you* stand in the spotlight.

    Congratulations! You have completed Day #2, and I hope you didn't have to break a sweat to come up with your affair. Let's get ready for your time to shine!

Day #3

Timeline for Your Affair

We are making great progress! You have determined that you *will* have an affair and you have set a date for the affair to take place. Your assignment for Day #3 is to determine your timeline and why this affair is important to you.

Simply put, your timeline for your affair is the amount of time you are willing to commit to reaching your goals. When I was preparing for the Miss Fitness Universe Pageant, I set my timeline based on the event's date. Then, I looked at my starting date—the date I was formally committing to preparing for my affair. I counted the weeks I had to complete my goals. This sharpened my focus toward being successful. After all, where is the fun in having an affair and not enjoying it?

Now, Day #3 is all about determining the amount of time available to you to reach your goals before the affair will take place. Be sure to be thorough in your research of the affair. Consider travel time to and from the affair, pre-affair meetings, and other considerations. Your affair does not have to take place prior to you completing this *Fit Happens Journal*, but I want to make sure you have enough time to take action and realize success using your *Fit Happens Journal*.

Items Needed

Pencil/Pen
Calendar

Now that you have an affair, you have to determine when the affair will take place.
In the space provided here, please write down the date of the affair.

My affair will take place on:

_____

(Date of the Affair)

Number of weeks to complete my affair:

_____

(Count the number of weeks from today's date)

Day #4

Importance of Your Affair

Do you remember my earlier question? Did you choose an affair that is good for you or good for someone else? Be sure to base your affair (goal) on what you want because you will be the one working hard to reach your personal target.

The importance of your affair has a great deal to do with the significance of the event. Any type of competitive event (pageants, marathons, or recitals, for example) puts you, your skills, and your talent in the spotlight. All eyes will be on you and on every part of your exterior! A family reunion or a special vacation are both wonderful opportunities to connect with loved ones and get caught up on family life and personal details. The bottom line is your affair should be memorable because of your connection to the people involved and the good feelings you receive from those connections. How you look when you're engaged in your affair should enhance those good feelings, not cause stress or feelings of inadequacy.

Items Needed

Pen/Pencil
Honest Opinion

In your own words, please write down why your affair (goal) is important to you. What does it mean to you to reach your goal? What would/could happen to you if you do not reach your goal?

_____

_____

_____

_____

_____

Day #5

Whom Are You Listening to Right Now?

Day #5 is the time to take a closer look at who has your ear—that is, whom do you listen to on a regular basis ... especially right now? Do you really know who's in your corner? Have you really thought about it?

When I set a goal and truly commit to achieving it, I will surround myself with people, places, and things that will help me reach my goals. The people who help me achieve them are my husband, my extended family, and a few special friends. I have been blessed to be surrounded by positive, uplifting people, and their support is both natural and genuine. The places are determined by the goal I have in mind or the affair on which I've set my sights.

For the sake of health and wellness, my favorite places to go when I'm working on a healthier lifestyle are gyms, fitness centers, and venues where healthy food choices are served. My things are motivational CDs, DVDs, and inspirational downloads. I constantly listen to motivational speakers while I work out, drive my car, clean the house, etc. I can always multi-task and feed my mind with motivational thoughts.

Your To-Do List for Day #5 is to answer the question, "Who Has Your Ear?" Please devote some serious thought to the following lists.

This exercise will help you build your support base. It's vital to surround yourself with encouraging voices speaking the language of inspiration and hope.

Items Needed

Pen/Pencil
Honest Thoughts

People

_____

_____

(Please list the people in your life who will help you reach your goal.)

Places

_____

_____

(Please list the places you can go that will help you reach your goal.)

Things

_____

_____

(Please list the things in your life that will help you reach your goal.)

Day #6

Quotes to Live By

Are you asking yourself, "Where is all of this going?" It's Day #6 and we haven't even started preparing to run a marathon or working on dropping ten pounds in a week. Well, that's not a part of this program! The philosophy in place here is to help you take a closer look at your environment and assess your passion and your willingness to take a step in a healthier direction. Flip back to Day #1. You have to remember that Day #1 did not happen overnight, nor will your affair happen overnight. Together we are going to work extremely hard to make changes that can last you a lifetime.

Okay, I'm stepping off my soapbox; let's focus on Day #6. I would like to know if you have an all-time favorite quote, saying, or scripture that motivates you. Have you heard of a famous "quote to live by" recently? Are you motivated by words? Only you can answer those questions.

I am motivated by quotes! I love quotes because I can always rely on them to encourage me when I may feel like giving up on my goal. My original quote to live by is the following:

Today is a New Day!
I will choose Success over Failure
Strength over Weakness!

I will Love my Body Nutritionally
Not Harm it Carelessly
Because Today is a New Day!

Your To-Do List for Day #6 is to create your own quote. Write down a positive thought or phrase that will keep you focused on your goal. The key to writing a motivational thought is that it should be positive as well as meaningful. It should not be negative. It serves to lift you up, not threaten you or to tear you down.

Please give this a lot of thought; you will rely on your own words in a later portion of this *Fit Happens Journal.*

Items Needed

Pen/Pencil

Motivational Thoughts

_____

_____

_____

_____

_____

(Think of what motivates you.)

Day #7

Day of Reflection and Giving

Hooray! You have successfully made it through Week #1. Today is a day of reflection and giving. At every step on this journey, it's necessary to maintain your focus on reaching your goal. It's essential that you understand the ultimate change that will happen when you do! That's right ... *when* and not *if*!

Reflection comes in realizing how far you've come and being thankful for the journey. You didn't have to pick up this guide, but I'm so glad you did. You've made a conscious, positive decision to pursue a healthier lifestyle, not just to drop a few pounds with the latest diet craze. Taking the time to genuinely evaluate leaving old habits behind and making the mental space for new, healthy behavior is one of the best ways to give you a mental lift.

Speaking of giving, this is your opportunity to give something back on multiple levels. Flip back to Day #5 and consider:

- calling one of the people who keeps you motivated and say a word of thanks,
- sharing one of your favorite places with a friend you haven't spoken to in a while, or
- doing one of the things on your list for someone else as a secret surprise.

Whatever you do, enjoy your day and be thankful for all the positive changes that are headed your way!

Items Needed

Pen/Pencil
Giving Heart

To-Do List for Day #7:

- Return to Day #1 and read everything in this *Fit Happens Journal* from that page to this page. Keep an open mind about what you have written on every page.
- Take a close look at the affair you want to have and what it would mean to you to reach that affair or goal.
- Look at your picture from Day #1 and ask yourself, "Am I happy with the person I see there?"
- Re-evaluate your current surroundings according to the people, places, and things listed on Day #5. Look at who and what surrounds your life today.

Now, here's what I want you to do: put down this *Fit Happens Journal* and reach out to someone who has shared his or her goals with you. No matter what goal the individual is pursuing, reach out and support that person's efforts. If you feel as though you can contribute to that person's ability to reach a higher level of achievement, or a more positive outlook, go for it! Choose your giving wisely. Be sincere. You will be surprised at how helping others can really help you in the end.

Use the following page to take notes from Week #1. I look forward to our journey tomorrow when we kick off Week #2!

Recap Your Week

Lessons Learned:

_____
_____
_____
_____

To-Do List:

_____
_____
_____
_____

Notes:

_____
_____
_____
_____

Week Two

Nutrition

Day #8

What Are You Eating?

Alright! You came back for more! The *Fit Happens Journal* is designed to help you get fit and stay fit. Have you noticed I still haven't mentioned anything about losing weight? Generally, when you lose something, you want to find it again. When I want to get healthy, I surround myself with the tools I need to help me reach my goals.

How do you know what tools are needed to get fit? Only you can really decide, but I want to share a few tools for you to consider. I surround myself with clean, natural, whole foods. My pantry and refrigerator are filled with fresh fruits and vegetables, whole grain breads, fresh dairy products, foods containing healthy oils and zero trans fats, and lean protein.

If you have any questions about any of these items, be sure to research all food groups for yourself. As a reminder, I will refer to or include examples of the strict eating plan I have used when preparing for both figure competitions and pageants. The foods listed are not federally endorsed have not been tested for diagnosis, treatment, or prevention of any diseases. Please consult your doctor before starting, changing, or altering your eating program.

Everyone's nutritional needs vary. It is dependent on, but not limited to, your age, health, gender, and other personal factors. For the sake of the *Fit Happens Journal,* I will keep it simple. If you want to educate yourself about the various food groups, and access some great tips and resources, please visit this link: www.MyPyramid.gov.

For Day #8, I want you to write down your favorite foods. Please answer the questions on the following page as honestly as possible. Use an additional page if necessary. Only you will know if you are telling the truth. I will not ask you to submit this journal when you complete it or ask you to give a formal presentation on its contents. This exercise will help you assess the nutritional content of the food you're eating and determine if those items are helping you reach your fitness goals.

Items needed

Pencil/Pen
Access to Kitchen and/or Pantry

Please list your favorite foods:

Breakfast—Whether it is fast food or your favorite cooked meal
My Snacks—Items you grab on the go or when you are watching TV
Lunch—Fast food, restaurant-based, home-cooked leftovers, or a sandwich from home—just write it down
Dinner—Fast food, restaurant-based, home-cooked leftovers, or a sandwich from home—sound familiar?
Dessert—What you cannot live without
Drink—What you drink most often

Meals	Items You Eat	Quantity Eaten
Breakfast		
My Snacks		
Lunch		
Dinner		
Dessert		
Drink		

Day #9

What Are You Eating?
Part II

For Day #9 take inventory of what you currently have in your home to eat. Answer the questions on the following page as honestly as possible. Feel free to use an additional page if necessary. Again, I want to emphasize that only you will know if you are telling the truth. We're still trying to get a solid understanding of the food you like to eat and its nutritional content.

The list on the next page is based on items found on the USDA's MyPyramid Web site. I have provided a brief description of each food group as a resource for the next three days. I'm not trying to make you feel guilty about what you're eating. Please just write down what you eat on average—the types of foods rather than quantities—as accurately as possible. I promise it will all make more sense later in the *Fit Happens Journal.*

Items needed

Pencil/Pen
Access to Kitchen and/or Pantry

Meat and Beans—All foods containing meat, such as poultry or fish, and including dry beans or peas, eggs, nuts, and seeds.

Grains—Any food made from wheat, rice, oats, cornmeal, barley, or another cereal grain is a grain product. Bread, pasta, oatmeal, breakfast cereals, tortillas, and grits are examples of grain products.

Remember: just write down the types of food you eat in each category, and don't worry about the quantity.

Meat	Beans	Grains

Day #10

What Are You Eating?
Part III

You've made it to Day #10 and you're making excellent progress! This is the last day of taking inventory of what you currently have in your home to eat. Please fill out the table on the following page, similar to the one you completed on Day #9.

The list on the next page is based on items from the MyPyramid Web site. I have provided a brief description of each food group as a resource for your use in today's assignment.

Items needed

Pencil/Pen
Access to Kitchen and/or Pantry

Vegetables—These foods count as a member of the vegetable group, such as greens (mustard, collard, turnip, etc.), broccoli, tomatoes, kale, cucumbers, carrots, okra, beans, peas, and potatoes, for instance. Vegetables may be raw or cooked, fresh, frozen, canned, or dried/dehydrated and may be whole, cut-up, or mashed.

Fruit—Any fruit counts as part of the fruit group, including apples, oranges, peaches, pears, plums, nectarines, bananas, blueberries, grapes, etc. Fruits may be fresh, canned, frozen or dried and may be whole, cut-up, or pureed.

Dairy—All fluid milk products and many foods made from milk are considered part of this food group. Foods made from milk that retain their calcium content are part of the group, while foods made from milk that have little to no calcium, such as cream cheese, cream, and butter, should be counted in the Oils and Fats group. Most milk group choices should be fat-free or low fat.

Oils and Fats—List all oils and fats that are liquid at room temperature (like vegetable oils used in cooking), as well as oils and fats that are solid (such as butter, shortening, and lard). Oils come from many different plants, fish, and nuts. Be sure to list them all.

Vegetables	Fruit	Dairy	Oils and Fats

Day # 11

What Are You Really Eating?

Where exactly does a cream-filled cookie come from? Do you read the Nutrition Facts food labels when you shop? Since 1994, the FDA has required food labels called Nutrition Facts to be placed on most food packages, boxes, and outer wrappers. These labels are easy to find, ~~as they~~ and are usually located right next to the ingredients list.

Understanding how your food is packed and being aware of the expiration date are also very important. Also, figuring out how to read the food label itself is a priority. In order to make healthy decisions when you're walking the grocery aisles, you need to understand all the information on every label.

The Nutrition Facts Food Label

Nutrition Facts labels may be formatted vertically or horizontally on some packages, and small packages may feature an abbreviated version. Most often, you will find vertical Nutrition Facts food labels. For example, this is a food label like one you would see on a can of condensed chicken noodle soup.

Chicken Noodle Soup

Nutrition Facts

Serving Size 1/2 cup (120 ml) condensed soup
Servings Per Container about 2.5

Amount Per Serving

Calories 60	Calories from Fat 15

% Daily Value*

Total Fat 1.5g	**2%**
Saturated Fat 0.5g	**3%**
Trans Fat 0g	
Cholesterol 15mg	
Sodium 890gm	**37%**
Total Carbohydrate 8g	**3%**
Dietary Fiber 1g	**4%**
Sugars 1g	
Protein 3g	

Vitamin A	4%	**Calcium**	0%
Vitamin C	0%	**Iron**	2%

*Percent Daily Values are based on a 2,000 calorie diet.
Your Daily Values may be higher or lower depending on
your calorie needs.

	Calories	2000	2500
Total Fat	Less than	65g	80g
Sat Fat	Less than	20g	25g
Cholesterol	Less than	300mg	300mg
Sodium	Less than	2,400m	2400mg
Total Carbohydrate		300g	375g
Dietary Fiber		25g	30g

Food Label

Nutrition Facts—Serving Information

The top half of the Nutrition Facts label gives you serving information. The serving information shows the serving size and the number of servings contained in the product. This is key, because the information that you learn from the rest of the label depends on the serving size. There are two parts to the actual package size; this is not the same as the serving size and can be very misleading. If a package of cookies contains six cookies and a serving size is equal to two cookies, then the entire package contains three servings, not one. On the chicken noodle soup example here, it is important to note that a serving is one-half cup of the condensed soup, as it is served directly from the can and not one-half cup of the soup *after* water has been added. Always look at the Nutrition Facts label to see if the serving size should be measured or counted *before* the product is prepared or *after* preparation.

Nutrition Facts—Calories, Fat, Carbohydrates, and Protein

The next section of the Nutrition Facts food label contains information about calories, fat content, amount and types of carbohydrates, and amount of protein. The label shows the amounts in grams (g) or milligrams (mg), and it shows us the percentage of the daily total value needed for each of these nutrients. This is based on a 2,000 calorie per day diet. While it won't be exactly right for everybody, the percentage will give you an idea of how the food item will fit into an average nutritional plan.

Day # 11
What Are You Really Eating?

For Day #11, flip back to look at your favorite foods from Day #8. Based on your favorite foods, pick the three most common items you eat on a daily or weekly basis and refer to the labels on each item to fill in the following chart. By doing this, you will have a better understanding of what you are really eating. Here is the example of the Nutrition Facts label for Chicken Noodle Soup as your guide.

Items Needed

Pen/Pencil
Lists from Days #8, #9, and #10

Food Labels of three Regularly Eaten Items

Chicken Noodle Soup
Nutrition Facts
Serving Size 1/2 cup (120 ml) condensed soup
Servings Per Container about 2.5
Amount Per Serving
Calories 60   Calories from Fat 15
% Daily Value*
Total Fat 1.5g   2%
Saturated Fat 0.5g   3%
Trans Fat 0g
Cholesterol 15mg
Sodium 890gm   37%
Total Carbohydrate 8g   3%
Dietary Fiber 1g   4%
Sugars 1g
Protein 3g
Vitamin A 4%   Calcium 0%
Vitamin C 0%   Iron 2%

Food Label

Items:	(1)	(2)	(3)
Calories:			
Total Fat:			
Total Sodium:			
Total Carbohydrate:			
Protein:			
Quantity Consumed:			

Congratulations! You've made it through the hardest part—that is, understanding the content of what you are eating.

Day #12

Ready, Set, Eat!

Welcome to Day #12, and, no, we are not off to the races! Now that you've taken note of the food you eat and its overall content, it's time to take stock of *when* you are eating.

Just for today, we're going to take a twenty-four-hour snapshot of when you are eating during the day. A standard food diary would take into account a number of days; however, we're going for a quick view of today.

By filling out the following table, you will gain a clearer picture of your personal eating habits as you rock around the clock!

Items Needed

Pen/Pencil
Clock or watch

As you take note of the recorded times, include the instances when in-between-meal snacks happen to occur today. If you can't remember everything, that's fine. We're looking for a quick view of when your meals are taking place. Please note: this food diary also appears in the Appendix.

Meals	Items Eaten	Time of Day
Breakfast		
My Snacks		
Lunch		
My Snacks		
Dinner		
Drink	(quantity in ounces)	

Day #13

Let's Go Shopping!

On Day #13, let's have a little fun and take the *Fit Happens Journal* on the road ... and into the grocery cart! Today's assignment is to go shopping for a healthy item that you haven't tried before and incorporate it into one of your meals for today. For example, if you noticed that your favorite foods from Day #8 don't include many fresh fruits, write down and commit to purchasing a bag of fresh grapes or a container of juicy blueberries that you can munch on throughout the day as one of your in-between-meal snacks.

Sounds easy, right? Yes, it is! As always, we want to stick with a thoughtful approach to pursuing a healthy lifestyle. Think about ways to add more nutritious food choices to your diet. Take the initiative to actually add them. It will make a tremendous difference.

Items Needed

Pen/Pencil
This Journal

It's time to go shopping! In the space provided, write down a few food items that you'd like to try or want to eat more often. The-my snacks column-is for you to write down items you would like to eat for your snacks. This column will have items that also appear in other columns (example: blueberries would appear in the fruit and my snacks column). Please note: this shopping list also appears in the Appendix. When you are ready to head to the store, make certain you're going first thing in the morning and after you've eaten a small meal or a snack. Never go to the grocery store when you're hungry. Try to resist the samples waiting at the end of the aisles!

Meat/ Beans	Grains	Vegetables	Fruit	Dairy	Fats and Oils	My Snacks

Day #14

Day of Reflection and Giving

Three cheers for you! This is a milestone day and you should pat yourself on the back. This week involved a lot of thought, reading, and paying attention to details. When you are under the blazing spotlight of your affair, believe me, it will seem as if every detail of your entire being is up for inspection and review. This week's process follows the same idea—every area of your nutritional life has to be reviewed, assessed, and understood. The food we eat is the foundation of our strength and ability to accomplish our dreams and goals.

On Day #14, the reflection should be on the food you eat ... not just on what you eat but on *why* you eat it. Is it a dish with family history? Is it a snack you always have when you need a pick-me-up? Is it a special meal you cook when it's time to celebrate?

For today's exercise in giving, think about the ways you can "feed" someone else—feed them a word of encouragement, feed them your gratitude for their friendship, or feed a complete stranger with your smile. Consider extending your action to giving back to a homeless shelter, soup kitchen, or food pantry in your community. Donating your time as well as the cost of your favorite dish will go a long way toward feeding your own spirit!

Now, let's get ready for a tremendous Week #3!

Items Needed

Pen/Pencil
This Journal

What is your favorite food? Do you remember the first time you had your favorite food? Was it a special occasion or your family's tradition? Is it a way to treat yourself for a bad day? What is the trigger for your favorite food? Write it down.

_____

_____

_____

_____

In the space provided, write down your giving ideas about "feeding" someone else: would you feed them a word of encouragement, feed them your gratitude for their friendship, or feed a complete stranger with your smile? Even consider ideas about extending your action to giving back to a homeless shelter, soup kitchen, or food pantry in your community. Donating your time and maybe the cost of your favorite dish will go a long way toward feeding your own spirit! What would you do to feed someone else's spirit?

_____

_____

_____

_____

Recap Your Week

Lessons Learned:

_____
_____
_____
_____

To-Do List:

_____
_____
_____
_____

Notes:

_____
_____
_____
_____

Week Three

Exercise

Day # 15

Exercise Inventory

Today is a New Day!
I will choose Success over Failure
Strength over Weakness!
I will Love my Body Nutritionally
Not harm it Carelessly
Because Today is a New Day!

Hello, Healthy You! It is so good to see that you are continuing with your *Fit Happens Journal.* Please feel free to reflect on Weeks #1 and #2 if you need a refresher on any topics discussed. Reviewing Day #1 is another great way to stay motivated.

If you noticed, I started you with my motivational quote. Feel free to start your day with this quote or your original quote from Day #6. By doing this, you will automatically start your day with a positive mind-set.

Week #1 was spent looking at what was surrounding you emotionally and physically, and in Week #2 we reviewed the food you are eating (more about this on Day #22). For Week #3, I want us to focus on your surroundings in reference to exercise equipment, videos, and workout clothing. That's not the sum total of the week, so I'm not letting you off the hook that easily! We're going to combine Week #3's exercise inventory with all of the activities from Week #1.

Take a look around your residence. Don't forget to look in your closets, garage, attic, the trunk of your car, basement, or outdoor storage unit. I want you to take inventory of every piece of exercise equipment you currently own, every exercise video or DVD on your shelves and or stuffed into drawers, and all the workout clothing and athletic shoes you have, whether you use them or not.

Use the worksheet to list all of the items you found. Be sure to check under the bed, too!

Items Needed

Pen/Pencil
Access to all of your home's closets, drawers, storage spaces, etc.
Dust Cloth (maybe)

Check-list (√)	Exercise Equipment	Check-list (√)	Exercise Videos (full body and areas of focus)	Check-list (√)	Workout Clothes
	Treadmill		Abs		# of Shorts
	Bike (Recumbent)		Thighs		# of Pants
	Bike (Stationary)		Arms		# of T-Shirts
	Elliptical		Butt		# of Tank Tops
	Weights (lbs)		Legs		# of Socks
	Weights (lbs)		Full Body		# of Tennis Shoes
	Exercise Ball		Aerobic		# of Gym Bags
	Resistance Bands		Other		Other
	Resistance Rings				
	Jump Rope				
	Pedometer				
	Other				
	Other				

Gym Membership
Name of gym _____
Distance from gym to your residence (in miles) _____

Day # 16

One Mile Workout

Let's see ... you've inventoried all of your exercise equipment, as well as your videos and DVDs, clothing, and shoes. Now what, you may ask, will happen next? For Day #16 we are going to determine how long it takes you to complete one mile.

If you have a treadmill in your inventory (and it still works), check to see if it will track distance. If not, read the "One Mile Test—No Equipment" section. If your treadmill will track the distance for you, go directly to the "Pace" section.

One Mile Test – No Equipment

You can determine one mile a number of ways if you do not have equipment. You can travel to your local park or high school. Most parks will have a walking trail with the distance posted along the path, and high schools will generally have a track that is standard in size. If so, four laps are equivalent to one mile on the school's track. You can also visit your favorite mall and ask customer service about the walking distances between anchor stores.

You can also determine a one mile distance by driving in your car. Start from your driveway and reset your car's odometer to zero, then drive a path that you would feel comfortable walking. Once your car's odometer reaches a half mile (or states 0.50), you have reached a half-mile point. Try to take note of a landmark, natural or man-made. You've just learned the distance from your front door to that half-mile point. Now, turn around, return to your starting point and walk the route you've just learned.

Pace

During today's workout, determine the time it takes you to complete one mile of walking (or jogging if you are currently exercising on a regular basis). Remember you should consult a doctor prior to starting any exercise routine. Use a stopwatch, cell phone, or any other timekeeping device to track your time. By doing this exercise, you will have a baseline for monitoring your current fitness level. This is not a race. It is a way to see where you are physically. Stay with me here: the further you progress in this program, the more this baseline test will make sense to you.

Be sure to pace yourself. This is the way for you to see the two important things from today's work: first, you can complete the workout; second, you can actively utilize the exercise tools you already own or resources readily available to you.

Items Needed

Pen/Pencil
This Journal
Timing Device (Stopwatch, clock, other)
Exercise Clothes
Access to Treadmill or Outdoors
Can-do Attitude

Equipment Used for Determining One Mile (Place a √ by your choice)
Treadmill
Outdoors
Other
Local Park
Local School Track
Route inside the Mall

Today's Date: _____

Your Time: _____

I completed one mile by
Walking
Jogging
Crawling
By a Miracle

Now I feel (please list your emotions)

_____
_____
_____
_____

The last time I did that much exercise was (date or year). _____

Day #17

Exercise Video Workout

Today is a New Day!
I will choose Success over Failure
Strength over Weakness!
I will Love my Body Nutritionally
Not harm it Carelessly
Because Today is a New Day!

Way to go! You made it through the one mile workout. Now I have a new workout option for you. Guess what? You get to stay indoors for this exercise. Please look back at Day #15's Inventory Sheet. Dust off your exercise videos and remind yourself why you bought them. Exercise videos are a great way to get a workout without leaving your home.

Regardless of which video you have or the series you own, please locate the video that will give you a full body workout. If it does not state what type of workout it is, make sure it features at least twenty-five minutes of movement and incorporates a workout for your legs. Videos that are formulated for "Abs Only" or "Arms Only" will not work. The key to Day #17 is to get your entire body moving, not just one body part. If you don't own a full body workout video, I recommend the *5 STEPS to a Healthier You* series, and you can find it on my Web site at www.StephanieSewell.com. You can locate something similar at your local public library.

Go ahead and move whatever furniture is in the way, queue up the video, and get started!

Items Needed

Pen/Pencil
Exercise Video
Exercise Clothes
Area to Exercise
Can-do Attitude

Name of Exercise Video _____

Length of Video _____

How do you feel physically prior to starting the exercise video? (Please write out your emotions.)

_____
_____
_____
_____

How do you feel physically now that you have completed the exercise video? (Please write out your emotions.)

_____
_____
_____
_____

Day # 18

One Mile Workout (One More Time!)

Here we go again! This week, you've successfully completed two days of exercise. I hope your response is "ready for more!" You've reached a major milestone on your journey to a healthier lifestyle. Now it is time to repeat Day #16. As a reminder, you can determine one mile any number of ways if you do not have equipment. You can travel to your local park, a high school track, or use a pedometer to keep track of your steps at the mall. Refer to the steps mentioned for Day #16.

Pace

During today's workout, determine the time it takes you to complete one mile. We want to see if you can maintain or improve your pace from Day #16.

You can use a stopwatch, cell phone, or any other timing device to track your time. By doing this exercise, you will have another baseline for monitoring your progress. Once again, the further you progress in this program, the more sense these exercises will make.

Be sure to pace yourself, and at the risk of sounding redundant, *this is not a race*. This is a way for you to see the same two things from

Day #16: first, you can complete the workout; second, you can use the exercise tools you already own or resources readily available to you.

Items Needed

Pen/Pencil
This Journal
Timing Device (stopwatch, clock, other)
Exercise Clothes
Access to Treadmill or Outdoors
Can-do Attitude

Equipment Used for Determining One Mile (Place a √ by your choice)
Treadmill
Outdoors
Other
Local Park
Local School Track
Route inside the Mall

Today's Date and Time of Day: _____

Your Time: _____

I completed the mile by

Walking
Jogging
Crawling
By a Miracle
Now I feel ... (Please list your emotions)

_____
_____
_____
_____

The last time I did that much exercise was (date or year) _____

Circle your choice:
The time today was (same, better, worse) than my time on Day #16.

Why do you think you had these results?

_____

_____

_____

_____

Day # 19

Exercise Video Workout (One More Round!)

Look at you! You've successfully completed three days of exercise. This is a crucial day, because you're probably starting to feel all those body parts in a new way! Keep reminding yourself that it's all a part of the journey to that healthier lifestyle. Now, it's time to repeat Day #17. As a reminder, you should use a video that will give you a full body workout. Refer to the steps mentioned for Day #17.

Although you should feel more comfortable with the pace and content of the video, try to complete the whole routine outlined on the video and don't forget to warm up with some light stretching and breathe this time.

Items Needed

Pen/Pencil
Exercise Video
Exercise Clothes
Area to Exercise
Can-do Attitude

Name of Exercise Video _____

Length of Video _____

How do you feel physically prior to starting the exercise video? (Please write out your emotions.)

_____
_____
_____
_____

How do you feel physically now that you have completed the exercise video? (Please write out your emotions.)

_____

Circle your choice:
My workout today was (same, better, worse) than my workout on Day #17.
Why do you think you had these results?

_____
_____
_____
_____

Day # 20

Hey D.J., Let's Mix Things Up!

Remember our discussion on Day #6? The *Fit Happens Journal*'s philosophy is to help you take a closer look at your surroundings and assess your desire and willingness to take a step in a healthier direction. In order to keep you motivated and focused, it is sometimes necessary to mix things up. On Day #20, your steps to a healthier lifestyle include a few dance steps as well as your own turn as the D.J.!

What handful of songs get your toes tapping and your fingers snapping? Scan your iPod's playlist for your favorite songs, or break out that CD player. You'll need to find five to seven songs that you can play back-to-back. You might enjoy these tunes so much you'll want to set the whole thing on repeat! That would be great, but we only need to accomplish one dance session with your selected songs.

The goal for Day #20 is to incorporate some movement that will keep you going for at least twenty-five minutes, just like with Days #16, #17, #18, and #19. If you choose the play list, then I know you'll enjoy your dance session. Hey, D.J., spin your best tunes, then show off your best moves!

Feel free to enjoy your favorite tunes while multi-tasking. You can "boogie" from room to room while cleaning the house, show off your fancy footwork on a dance floor, or dance with a loved one or family member in your living room. Whatever you choose, just have fun!

Items Needed

Pen/Pencil
Names of Five to Seven of Your Favorite Songs
Space to Dance
This Journal
Time Device (stopwatch, clock, etc.)
Can-do Attitude

Use the space provided to list your favorite songs by title and artist:

_____

_____

_____

_____

_____

_____

_____

Time you began your dance session:

_____

How do you feel physically prior to starting your dance session? (Please write out your emotions.)

_____

_____

_____

_____

Time you ended your dance session: _____

How do you feel physically now that you have completed your dance session? (Please write out your emotions.)

_____

_____

_____

_____

Day #21

Day of Reflection and Giving

Wow! Look at your progress! I'm so proud to welcome you to Day #21! You have accomplished so much, and we need to give thanks for your stamina! I thank you for sticking with the program because now we're ready to see the changes you've been making! I haven't forgotten about your affair, and I'm sure you haven't either.

There's plenty of reflection for today, and we'll focus on how you feel now that you've survived a week of exercise. Are you energized or tired? Did you feel "the burn" and were you able to work through it anyway? Has your opinion changed about exercising? Why or why not?

For today's giving exercise, let's think about what you're giving to yourself every time you exercise: toned muscles, stronger limbs, more oxygen in your lungs, and more endorphins (the "happy hormones") flowing through your body. You're doing so much good for yourself when you give your body the gift of exercise. Does it get any better than that? You bet it does, because here comes Week #4!

Items Needed

Pen/Pencil
This Journal

In the space provided, write down your reflections on the week of exercising. Are you energized or tired? Did you feel "the burn" and were you able to work through it anyway? Has your opinion changed about exercising? Why or why not? What was your favorite exercise this week?

_____

_____

_____

_____

In the space provided, write down the benefits you're "giving" to yourself every time you exercise. Do your muscles look more toned? Do your limbs feel stronger? Are you taking more deep breaths? What is the biggest change you've noticed? Did you notice more endorphins (the "happy hormones") flowing through your body? Did your loved ones, family, or friends notice a difference? Talk to them. Ask them!

_____

_____

_____

_____

Recap Your Week

Lessons Learned:

_____
_____
_____
_____

To-Do List:

_____
_____
_____
_____

Notes:

_____
_____
_____
_____

Week Four

Bringing It All Together

Day #22

Nutritious Breakfast and One Mile Workout

Congratulations! You made it to Week #4. This week, we are going to bring it all together. I want you to choose when you will exercise. Choose morning or evening— either is fine as long as you exercise.

Although this is the final week in the *Fit Happens Journal*, it is not your final week of progressing to a Healthier You! This is only the end of a great beginning. You must continue and complete this week. You wouldn't start a race and walk away before you reached the finish line, would you?

Also, the *Fit Happens Journal* was designed with you in mind. I wanted to take you step by step through the journey I take when I need to get healthier. Please be sure to work through Week #4 and complete this journey. I want you to have a feeling of accomplishment when you have your affair.

For Day #22, select a nutritious breakfast to start your day. My definition of a nutritious breakfast is food that is fresh and naturally colorful. If your breakfast comes from a bag or box, be sure to add something fresh and naturally colorful to it. Some examples I eat for my healthy breakfast are listed here. Be sure to choose foods you like while keeping in mind the fresh and naturally colorful options.

My favorites for breakfast are whole grain breads (I look for 100 percent whole grain content), oatmeal, fresh fruit, eggs, and lean protein such as turkey bacon or grilled chicken.

My very favorite nutritious breakfast is this:

½ cup of oatmeal
Omelet made with four egg whites and mushrooms, spinach, and low-fat mozzarella cheese
2 strips of turkey bacon
½ cup of fresh berries
20 ounces of water

Can you picture my mouth-watering, fresh and naturally colorful items on my breakfast menu? Now, it's your turn to select a nutritious breakfast for yourself.

Also, it's time to get you moving with the one mile workout. I told you we were going to bring it all together with this equation: Nutritious Eating + Exercising = a Healthier You. Let's get started.

Items Needed

Pen/Pencil
This Journal
Timing Device (stopwatch, clock, other)
Exercise Clothes
Access to Treadmill or Outdoors
Can-do Attitude
Nutritious Breakfast

Meals	Items Eaten	Time of Day
Breakfast		

Equipment Used for Determining One Mile (Place a √ by your choice)
Treadmill
Outdoors
Other
Local Park
Local School Track
Route inside the Mall

Today's Date and Time of Day _____

Your Time _____

I completed the mile by
Walking
Jogging
Crawling
By a Miracle

Now I feel ... (Please list your emotions.)

_____

_____

_____

_____

The last time I did that much exercise was (This *better* be the date of Day #18). _____

Day #23

Nutritious Breakfast, Lunch, and Exercise Video

Look at you! You've successfully completed Day #22. You started your day with a nutritious breakfast, and you completed your one mile workout, right? If you cannot answer that question honestly, please flip back to Day #22 and complete it before moving to this day. The only way this journal will work for you is if you are honest with yourself. If you need some motivation, flip back to Day #6 to refresh yourself with your quote to keep you on track.

Okay, now on Day #23, we are going to focus on having a nutritious lunch. I want you to repeat your nutritious breakfast for today as well as use your exercise video for your workout.

Personally, I like to use the same guidelines I shared with you for breakfast for all of my meals. I like for my meals to be (all together now!) *nutritious* by being fresh and naturally colorful.

My favorites for my healthy lunch are listed here. Be sure to choose foods you like while keeping in mind the fresh and naturally colorful options.

My lunch favorites include salads (with dark mixed green lettuce), whole grain breads (again, look for 100 percent whole grain content), lean turkey, fish, or grilled chicken and fresh fruit.

My favorite nutritious lunch is this one:

- 4-6 ounces grilled chicken on mixed greens with cucumbers, tomatoes, carrots, one sliced hard-boiled egg, and a sprinkle of low-fat mozzarella cheese, mixed with EVOO (extra virgin olive oil) and balsamic vinegar
- 1 medium-sized apple
- 20 ounces of water

Can you picture my delicious lunch of fresh and naturally colorful items? Now, it's your turn to select a nutritious lunch for yourself.

Don't forget to exercise! You can determine whether to complete your exercise video in the morning or evening, as long as you do it. As a reminder, you should use a video that will give you a full body workout. Check through your collection of videos that you inventoried on Day #15. I hope you feel more comfortable with the pace and content of the video you have selected for today. I encourage you to continue to try to complete the whole routine outlined on the video. First, warm up with some light stretching and continue to breathe.

Items Needed

Pen/Pencil
Exercise Video
Exercise Clothes
Area to Exercise
Can-do Attitude

Meals	Items Eaten	Time of Day
Breakfast		
Lunch		

Name of Exercise Video _____
Length of Video _____

How do you feel physically prior to starting the exercise video? (Please write out your emotions.)

_____

_____

_____

_____

How do you feel physically now that you have completed the exercise video? (Please write out your emotions.)

_____

Circle your choice:

My workout today was (same, better, worse) than my workout on Day #19.

Why do you think you had these results?

_____

_____

_____

_____

Day #24

Nutritious Breakfast, Lunch, Snacks, and Dinner

Wow! You are amazing! You are determined to complete this four-week journal and continue on your journey to a Healthier You! I'm so excited for you!

Today, we are going to focus on a full day of healthy eating. This is the second time in the journal I am asking you to write down everything you eat throughout the day. Then, and only then, I want you to turn back to Day #12 to compare the items you listed today with Day #12's items. Are you eating the same types of food? I hope not, especially if you were eating non-nutritious foods at the beginning of this journey.

We have discussed nutritious breakfast and lunch items. Now, we will focus on nutritious snacks and dinner items. I will continue to reference the same guidelines I shared with you for breakfast, lunch, and for all of my meals. I like my meals to be nutritious by being fresh and naturally colorful (sound familiar?).

I really want to drive this point home. When you eat naturally colorful foods, you are generally eating foods in their natural state. Examples include delicious red apples, juicy green grapes, golden grapefruit, crisp orange carrots, fresh green cucumbers, and the list can go on and on. All of these items are great snacks. Choose one of them or find your favorite, fresh vegetable or fruit as your snack today. Eat one between your breakfast and lunch and choose another one as your snack between lunch and dinner.

Some examples I eat for a nutritious snack include these:

- 1 cup of celery sticks with 2 tablespoons of hummus
- ½ large grapefruit
- 1 cup carrots with low-fat ranch veggie dip

My favorite items I like to eat for dinner are these:

- Grilled or broiled chicken or fish, salads, vegetables, whole grain rice, or a baked sweet potato.

My favorite nutritious dinner is this one:

- 4–6 ounces of broiled salmon
- ½ baked sweet potato
- Mixed green salad with EVOO (extra virgin olive oil) and balsamic vinegar
- 20 ounces of water

Now, it is your turn to select your nutritious foods for today. It is best to plan your entire day, just like you plan your wardrobe according to the weather or occasion. Happy eating!

Items Needed

Pen/Pencil
This Journal

Meals	Items Eaten	Time of Day
Breakfast		
My Snacks		
Lunch		
My Snacks		
Dinner		
Drink	(quantity in ounces)	

Day #25

Nutritious Breakfast, Lunch, Snacks, Dinner, and Exercise

Can you see the goal line? You're almost there! For Day #25, we are bringing it all together. Today is the first day of a brand new you. By completing every challenge, including today's, you have successfully learned and implemented the key to reaching your goals.

Nutritious eating and regular exercise lead to a Healthier You!

This is a crucial day. Even though we did not emphasize exercise on Day #24, you are probably starting to feel those body parts you have been exercising in a completely different way! Keep reminding yourself that it's all part of the journey to that healthier lifestyle.

For Day #25, I want you to repeat everything you have learned. You should repeat your nutritious breakfast, snack, lunch, snack, and dinner plan, as well as find time either in the morning or evening to complete your One Mile Workout. You're doing this because … Today is a New Day! I will choose Success over Failure … Strength over Weakness! I will Love my Body Nutritionally … Not Harm it Carelessly … Because Today is a New Day!

Meals	Items Eaten	Time of Day
Breakfast		
My Snacks		
Lunch		
My Snacks		
Dinner		
Drink	(quantity in ounces)	

Please note: this food diary also appears in the Appendix.

Items Needed

Pen/Pencil
This Journal
Timing Device (stopwatch, clock, other)
Exercise Clothes
Access to Treadmill or Outdoors
Can-do Attitude

Equipment Used for Determining One Mile (Place a √ by your choice)
Treadmill
Outdoors
Other
Local Park
Local School Track
Route inside the Mall

Today's Date and Time of Day _____

Your Time _____

I completed the mile by
Walking
Jogging
Crawling
By a Miracle

Now I feel ... (Please list your emotions.)

_____
_____
_____
_____

The last time I did that much exercise was (I hope this is the date of Day #22). _____

Day #26

You Make Me Feel Like Dancing!

How do you feel? I hope the answer is "Great!" I am ecstatic you are reading and ready to complete Day #26. You have achieved so much during this journey to a Healthier You. You have completed more than four miles of walking and/or jogging, danced to your own favorite tunes, worked up a sweat with your favorite exercise videos, and you are eating nutritious foods—foods that are good for your mind, body, and mood. You make me feel like celebrating and dancing. Hey! Why don't we do just that? Let's party tonight!

For Day #26, I want you to continue to eat nutritiously fresh, naturally colorful foods for breakfast, lunch, and your two snacks. Look back over the items you have been eating for Week #4 as a guide. For dinner, I want you to find a restaurant that offers healthful choices.

Many of the famous chain restaurants will have entrée items listed on their website with their nutrition content. Research a restaurant in your area; it may be your personal favorite or one you have been eager to try. Just make sure there are healthy choices to select from on the menu.

I would like to share some guidelines I use when eating out:

- Ask the server to hold the bread for the table.
- Ask for water to drink.
- Ask the server for examples of the portion sizes for appetizers and entrées.
- Skip the fried foods and desserts.
- Leave a good tip (due to all of the questions).

After you have enjoyed your restaurant of choice, I would like you to go dancing! I'm sure you are thinking, *"Dancing right after eating? Who would do that?"* You would, and you can because you controlled your meal portions and now you are ready to hit the dance floor!

You may choose to visit a dance club, or you may head home for a fun night of dancing around the house! All I ask is that you are grooving to the music like you did on Day #20. This is a time to celebrate the fact that you are a healthier person and you have completed the *Fit Happens Journal*. Even though we have two more days left in the journal, you have completed the toughest part.

Now, get moving and start researching your restaurant choices!

Items Needed

Pen/Pencil
This Journal
Web site or Restaurant Guide
Dancing Shoes

My Tips for Eating Out:
- Hold the bread for the table.
- Ask for water as your beverage.
- Clarify the portion sizes for appetizers and entrées.
- Skip the fried foods and desserts.
- Leave a good tip (if possible).

Restaurant: _____
Nutrition Information of Menu Items Selected:

_____

_____

_____

_____

Did you do the following?
Hold the bread for the table
Water for your drink
Clarify portion sizes for appetizers and entrées
Skip the fried foods and desserts
Leave a good tip, if possible

Grade Yourself on Eating Out _____
- A-Accomplished your goal
- B-Bit off a little too much to chew (almost overdid it)
- F-Failed miserably

Day #27

Progress Check

I'm so glad you are completing the *Fit Happens Journal!* I'm glad to know that you are ready to see how far you've come from Day #1. In order to know the distance you have traveled, you have to know your personal starting point. Day #1 was all about you and so is Day #27. Welcome to your progress check!

For Day #27, have someone take your picture and measurements for you. I would recommend you wear something fitted and comfortable for this brief photo session. Try to find your original outfit from Day #1. Also, I still suggest having more skin showing in your picture.

When having your picture and measurements taken, resist the temptation to hold in your stomach! Do not hold your breath! Do not wear baggy clothes! And, whatever you do, *do not skip* Day #27. This is *now* the most important day!

It is time for you to see the new you! Trust me. My clients who opted to skip Day #1 in their Fit Happens journey were very unhappy about not documenting their starting point. So, since you did complete Day #1, let's go ahead and complete Day #27.

Items Needed

Pen/Pencil
Camera
Someone to Take Your Picture
Fitted Outfit
Measuring Tape
Scale

Date:
Weight:
Height:

Measurements (inches)
Neck:
Chest:
Waist (Circumference of Natural Curve):
Waist (Circumference from Belly Button):
Hips:
Upper Thigh (Widest Part):
Arm (Circumference of Bicep):

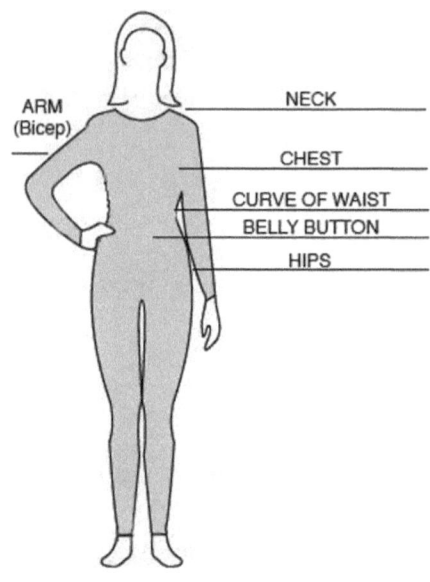

[Insert Photo Here]

Day #28

Day of Reflection and Giving

Congratulations! You have officially completed the *Fit Happens Journal.* How do you feel? What have you learned about yourself?

Let's reflect over the past week, as well as the past twenty-eight days. I would like you to compare Day #1 to Day #27.

Do you like what you see? _____

Can you tell a difference for the better? _____

Are you one step closer to having your affair? _____

Although Day #28 marks the end of our four weeks together, your journey does not stop here.

Please consider this journal your go-to resource for reinforcing your overall body confidence, encouraging positive, health-enhancing habits, and serving as your personal reminder of what *you* can accomplish when you have a solid plan in hand!

When you break it all down, this handbook spells out the solution to a Healthier You, and you can return at any time:

- Get Up: Being clear about your fitness goals is a conscious decision to be positive or "up" about your health!
- Get Moving: You can't accomplish any goal, fitness or otherwise,

by sitting on your rear. Burning calories requires sweat-inducing activity, and achieving goals requires movement.

- Get Fit: This is a dual commitment to eating nutritiously and maintaining an active interest in exercise. When you establish the habit, your body can't help but get hooked!

Your mind is your strongest ally in achieving your goal of living a healthier lifestyle. When you "know" the right way to shop and eat, the best ways to incorporate exercise into your day, and the exact way to keep yourself motivated, you are claiming success in the ongoing battle of the bulge, the war of the raging muffin top, and the fight against frightening love handles!

Fit Happens Program: If you're going to set a goal, it's important to create a plan that will help you succeed. The plan is your step-by-step guide that tells you what to do next and helps you stay encouraged and focused. I hope you've found a positive plan for success with this *Fit Happens Journal*! Remember:

Today is a New Day!
I will choose Success over Failure
Strength over Weakness!
I will Love my Body Nutritionally
Not Harm it Carelessly
Because Today is a New Day!

Items Needed

Pen/Pencil
This *Fit Happens Journal*

In the space provided, write down your reflections on Week #4. Are you energized or tired? Has your opinion changed about exercising and eating nutritiously? Why or why not? What was your favorite meal of the week?

_____

_____

_____

_____

Write down the benefits you're "giving" to yourself every time you exercise and eat healthfully. Do your muscles look more toned? Do your limbs feel stronger? Are you taking more deep breaths? What is the biggest change you've noticed? Did you notice more endorphins (the "happy hormones") flowing through your body? Did your loved ones, family, and friends notice a difference? Talk to them. Ask them!

_____

_____

_____

_____

Write your reflections on sharing one of your favorite nutritious meals with friends and family:

_____

_____

_____

_____

Recap Your Week

Lessons Learned:

_____
_____
_____
_____

To-Do List:

_____
_____
_____
_____

Notes:

_____
_____
_____
_____

About the Author

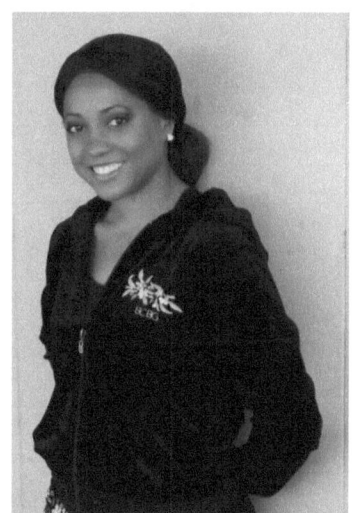

Stephanie Sewell, Certified Personal Trainer, Certified Group Fitness Instructor, and Certified Nutrition and Wellness Consultant, guides her clients through the *Fit Happens with Know Exercise: 28 Days of Success for Every Body (Fit Happens Journal)*. Whether her clients are absolute beginners or accomplished athletes, Stephanie inspires and motivates people to help them achieve and maintain their ideal body and weight. All they need is a "can-do" attitude to start, and they have completed her success journal and other exercise programs with flying colors!

Stephanie, an inaugural member of the NFL Carolina Panthers Cheerleading Squad, traveled to Hawaii to represent the team at the

ProBowl; she's a former pageant title holder (including swimsuit winner) and National Fitness/Figure/and Bikini Competitor. Stephanie knows firsthand the importance of documenting progress and believes it is the building block to slimming down and shaping up. Stephanie has designed this journal to share her secrets with you.

Visit StephanieSewell.com for these additional resources:

- *5 STEPS to a Healthier You*
- *5 STEPS to a Healthier You*—Kids Boot Camp Edition
- *Cardio in 5*—A four-disc audio cardiovascular workout program

Stay tuned for the next edition in the *Fit Happens with Know Exercise Journal* series.

Degree and Certifications

Stephanie obtained her BS degree from Western Carolina University. She is certified through American Fitness Professionals and Associates as an AFPA Certified Personal Trainer, AFPA Certified Group Fitness Instructor, and an AFPA Certified Nutrition and Wellness Consultant. She also works as a pharmaceutical representative specializing in diabetes care. She is a member of Toastmasters International and the National Speakers Association.

Competitive Accomplishments

- Miss Cherokee County (South Carolina) 1994
- Miss South Carolina America Swimsuit Preliminary Winner 1994
- Miss Spartanburg (South Carolina) USA 1997
- Miss South Carolina USA 3rd Runner Up 1997
- Miss Fitness America–ESPN Top 20 Finalist 1998
- NFL Carolina Panthers Cheerleader (1996) Co-Captain
- NFL Carolina Panthers Cheerleader (1997) Captain
- NFL Carolina Panthers Cheerleader (1998) TopCat of the Year
- NFL Carolina Panthers Cheerleader (1998) ProBowl Cheerleader
- National Bikini Competition Top 10 Finalist Classic Bikini and

- Model America 2006
- National Bikini and Figure Competition Top 10 Finalist Classic
- Bikini and Figure Universe 2009 (6th and 7th Place)
- National Physique Committee North America National Competition Masters Bikini and Open Bikini 4th Place
- National Physique Committee Jr. USA's National Competition Bikini Class B Winner

Shopping List

First shown on Day #13, this shopping list is a helpful resource for monitoring the types of food—and the nutrition content—you purchase from the grocery store.

Meat/ Beans	Grains	Vegetables	Fruit	Dairy	Fats and Oils	My Snacks

Food Diary

First shown on Day #12 and again on Day #25, this food diary is a helpful resource for tracking daily food consumption.

Meals	Items Eaten	Time of Day
Breakfast		
My Snacks		
Lunch		
My Snacks		
Dinner		
Drink	(quantity in ounces)	

www.ingramcontent.com/pod-product-compliance
Lightning Source LLC
Chambersburg PA
CBHW051442280526
45785CB00003B/1392